INTRAVENOUS TH...

A Guide to Basic Principles

Eugenia M. Fulcher, RN, BSN, MEd, EdD, CMA
Adjunct Instructor, Augusta Technical College
Waynesboro, Georgia

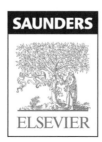

SAUNDERS

ELSEVIER

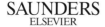

11830 Westline Industrial Drive
St. Louis, Missouri 63146

INTRAVENOUS THERAPY: A GUIDE TO BASIC PRINCIPLES   ISBN 10: 1-4160-3200-2
Copyright © 2006 by Saunders, an imprint of Elsevier Inc.   ISBN 13: 978-1-4160-3200-7

NOTICE

Knowledge and best practice in this field are constantly changing. Standard safety precautions must be followed, but as new research and clinical experience broaden our knowledge, changes in treatment and drug therapy may become necessary or appropriate. Readers are advised to check the most current product information provided by the manufacturer of each drug to be administered to verify the recommended dose, the method and duration of administration, and contraindications. It is the responsibility of the licensed prescriber, relying on experience and knowledge of the patient, to determine dosages and the best treatment for each individual patient. Neither the publisher nor the author assumes any liability for any injury and/or damage to persons or property arising from this publication.

ISBN 10: 1-4160-3200-2
ISBN 13: 978-1-4160-3200-7

Publisher: Michael S. Ledbetter
Developmental Editor: Celeste Clingan
Book Production Manager: Linda McKinley
Publishing Services Manager: Pat Joiner
Designer: Mark Oberkrom

Printed in the United States

Last digit is the print number: 9 8 7 6 5 4 3 2 1

Working together to grow
libraries in developing countries

www.elsevier.com | www.bookaid.org | www.sabre.org

ELSEVIER   BOOK AID International   Sabre Foundation

Introduction

This material is intended only as an introduction to the theory of IV therapy. The procedure for initiating and administering IV therapy requires that the practitioner have a working knowledge of the physiology of all body systems, understand fluid and electrolyte balance, and know the effects of medications and fluids on body systems. The three main categories of IV therapy outlined in this supplement are maintenance, restoration, and replacement, which is the most frequently performed. The actual procedure for starting IV therapy is discussed, but applying the mathematical concepts of IV therapy and performing the procedure also are necessary knowledge bases for patient safety.

IV therapy is not a basic medical assisting skill but an advanced skill to be practiced by medical assistants who have access to skilled health professionals knowledgeable in IV therapy. Medical assistants must always be aware of the expected scope of practice and the legal aspects of initiating IV therapy in their states of practice.

The basics of intravenous therapy

OBJECTIVES

At the completion of this material content, the student will be able to:

- Define the key terms associated with basic intravenous (IV) therapy
- Explain the physiology of fluids in maintaining homeostasis and electrolyte balance
- Describe the indications for and advantages of IV therapy
- Identify the dangers of IV therapy
- Identify the types of fluids used for IV replacement therapy
- List the factors used in determining the types of IV fluids used in therapy
- Identify the equipment and delivery systems needed for IV therapy
- Know the basic formulas for calculating drip rates for IV fluids
- Explain why the medical assistant must assess the patient and the related medical conditions before initiating IV therapy
- Discuss the legal and ethical issues of beginning IV therapy

GLOSSARY OF TERMS

Chemotherapy The use of chemicals to treat disease, usually cancer

Diuresis The increased excretion of urine

Drip chamber The elongated rigid section, located at the top of the tubing, that holds fluids for administration between the supply container and the tubing

Drop orifice The opening at the top of the drip chamber that determines the size and shape of the drop

Electrolytes A salt found in body tissues such as blood, tissue fluid, and cells; sodium, potassium, and chlorides are the most common electrolytes

Embolus, emboli Thrombus (thrombi), such as a blood clot, bone marrow, or air, that is moving through the vascular system

Extracellular fluids Body fluids found outside of the cell

Flow rate The rate at which IV fluids are regulated for administration

Hematoma A localized collection of blood, usually clotted, in an organ, a tissue, or a space

Homeostasis The balance of the internal environment of the body through feedback and responses when faced with external and internal changes

Hydrolysis The splitting of a compound into fragments by the addition of water

Hypertonic A solution that causes a flow of water out of the cell across its semipermeable membrane

Hypotonic A solution that causes the flow of water into the cell across its semipermeable membrane

Induration A raised, inflamed hardened area

Infiltration The leaking of IV fluid into surrounding tissue

Infusion therapy The therapeutic introduction of fluid other than blood into a vein

Interstitial fluids Fluids found between cells in the tissue layers

Interstitial spaces Spaces found between cells within tissue layers

Intracellular fluids Fluids within a cell

Isotonic A solution in which the body tissues can be bathed without the transfer of fluids across the semipermeable membrane of the cell

IV flush The washing out of an IV administration site with a fluid

IV therapy The introduction of therapeutic fluids directly into the venous circulation

Lethargy A lowered level of consciousness with listlessness, drowsiness, and apathy

Macrodrip Tubing that supplies large drops of fluids, such as 8 to 20 drops/mL

Metabolic acidosis A condition in which the acid-base status of the body shifts toward the acid side because of the loss of base elements or the retention of acids other than carbonic acid; opposite of respiratory acidosis

Metabolism The sum of all physical and chemical processes by which a living substance is produced and maintained and by which energy is made available for the uses of the organism

Metabolites Any substance produced by metabolism or by a metabolic process

Microdrip Tubing that supplies small drops of fluids, such as 60 drops/mL

Overload An excess amount of a substance in the body

Over-the-needle-catheter An infusion that uses a needle as a stylet and leaves a catheter in place for the infusion; the catheter is exterior to the needle

Parenteral The administration of a substance by injection

Phlebitis An inflammation of a vein

Plasma The fluid portion of blood

Replacement therapy Treatment to replace deficiencies in body substances by the administration of natural or synthetic substitutes

Respiratory acidosis A condition of acidosis that results from excess retention of carbon dioxide in the body; the opposite of metabolic acidosis, the condition is seen in chronic obstructive pulmonary disorder and other respiratory conditions that interfere with normal ventilation

Solute A substance, usually a solid material, that is dissolved in a solvent

Solvent A substance, usually a liquid, that dissolves or is capable of dissolving another substance

Thrombus, thrombi Stationary blood clot(s) along the wall of a blood vessel

Venous spasm A sudden but transitory constriction of a vein

Winged-infusion needle An infusion needle that has plastic holders on each side of the needle hub that help hold the needle in place during the injection

PHYSIOLOGY AND IV THERAPY

Water, accounting for approximately 60% to 75% of total body weight, is the single largest constituent of the body's mass and is essential to life. Fat cells contain less water, making the percentage of body water dependent on the fat distribution of the person. Age, gender, ethnic origin, and weight also are factors that influence the amount and distribution of body fluids.

Continually moving in the body, water is given different names in various locations, such an intracellular fluid, extracellular fluid, plasma, lymph, and interstitial fluid. Homeostasis depends on fluid and electrolyte intake and physiologic factors, disease processes, external factors, and pharmacologic interventions. Electrolytes for homeostasis are dissolved in the blood plasma, a body solvent, for transport throughout the body. Body fluids are continuously exchanged in the intracellular and interstitial spaces and plasma. For a person to remain in fluid homeostasis, that person must maintain an approximately equal intake to output of fluids.

Fluids function to maintain blood volume, regulate body temperature, and transport needed nutrients to and from cells for cell metabolism. Body fluids also aid in digestion through hydrolysis, act as a medium for excretion, and act as solvents in which the solutes are transported for cell function.

Body fluids contain 0.9% sodium chloride, and IV fluids are described as *isotonic* when they contain the same salt concentration as found in normal body fluids. For the person who needs only replacement of normally lost body fluids, isotonic fluids are used. Fluids that contain less salt (sodium chloride) than fluids found in the body are referred to as *hypotonic*. When hypotonic fluids are administered, the normal fluids in blood vessels shift from the circulating blood into the interstitial spaces and the interstitial tissue and cells. This actions hydrates cells but can deplete the circulatory system fluids. Hypertonic solutions contain greater concentrations of salt (sodium chloride) than those found in body fluids. Thus these solutions cause extracellular fluids to shift from the cells into the plasma in the blood. This action reduces body edema but increases the pressure in blood vessels, causing elevated blood pressure, hypertension, and increased work for the heart and lungs. Therefore the physician must carefully choose IV fluids to meet the specific needs of each person so that the body will remain in or quickly return to homeostasis. IV therapy has very specific indications and must be carefully chosen to meet the needs of the patient. The health professional who participates in IV therapy must be just as careful in preparing the order.

USES AND ADVANTAGES

For any medication to be effective, it must reach the blood for distribution throughout the body. Oral medications are absorbed through the digestive tract, and parenteral medications other than those given intravenously cross tissue barriers before absorption. With IV therapy, these barriers do not exist. The entire amount of medication is distributed in the bloodstream immediately after administration. Thus one of the major indications and advantages of IV therapy is the rapid absorption of medication.

For patients who are unable to take medication by mouth or for whom the ordered parenteral injection would cause irritation of tissues, such as with chemotherapy medications, the IV route is often indicated. When drugs are altered by the gastrointestinal tract to make the medication less effective, the preferred route also is parenteral. The preferred route is parenteral—perhaps specifically intravenously—in patients who are unconscious, vomiting, or uncooperative in oral intake.

The rationales for using IV therapy fall into three categories: maintenance therapy, replacement therapy, and restoration therapy. Each type of therapy has a specific rationale and a direct influence on the type of IV fluids ordered by the physician.

Maintenance therapy provides the necessary nutrients to meet the daily needs for water, electrolytes, and nutritional replacement. The amount of fluid is determined by the patient's age, height, weight, and amount of body fat. Maintenance therapy is used for patients who have either no intake of fluids by mouth or a very limited oral intake and require supplements of fluids and nutritional elements.

When a patient has had a deficit of fluids and electrolytes over time, usually 48 hours or more, **replacement therapy** may be needed. Patient indications include vomiting and diarrhea, starvation, and hemorrhage. Before replacement fluids are instituted, kidney function should be checked. Because of the increased volume of fluids added to the body and the inherent loss of potassium, potassium replacement also may be necessary to maintaining homeostasis.

Finally, **restorative therapy** is daily restoration of vital fluids and electrolytes. With this therapy, the fluids used are physiologically the same as the fluids being lost as determined by laboratory testing. Often several types of fluids are ordered for administration on the same day. This is more often seen in in-patient settings because of the dangers associated with fluid overload.

In an ambulatory care center, the most common type of IV therapy is replacement therapy. The allied health care professional responsible for the fluid IV administration should carefully monitor the person for any signs of overload or toxicity, such as increased blood pressure, breathing difficulties, chest discomfort, and other common symptoms of adverse reactions, such as itching, rashes, and edema.

THE DANGERS OF IV THERAPY

One obvious danger of IV therapy is the possible introduction of microorganisms directly into the bloodstream when aseptic technique is not precisely followed. Because fluids are introduced directly into the bloodstream for transport throughout the body, the strictest of aseptic techniques is necessary. Any possible loss of asepsis must be confronted and the equipment discarded to protect the patient. Sterility is not measured in degrees.

Another major danger is infection or inflammation at the injection site, including local infection and phlebitis. The care of the injection site and bandaging around the site must be performed using medical and surgical asepsis to prevent the spread of bacteria from the dressings to the vein through the injection site. Phlebitis at the site may result from IV fluid irritation, needle movement because of patient activity, and improper handling of fluids and equipment. The signs of phlebitis are discomfort and swelling and inflammation radiating from the administration site along the route of venous circulation.

The use of hypertonic or hypotonic solutions may cause destruction of blood cells, resulting in an embolus formation from the debris of these cells. Particles of undiluted medications that have not dissolved in the fluid also may result in an embolus. The person who administers the IV fluids must ensure that all medications have dissolved before beginning the IV therapy.

If the physician's order is not carefully followed or the fluids are given too rapidly and in large volumes over a short time, fluid overload of the body may occur. The circulatory system becomes overloaded with the excessive amounts of fluids. This condition is especially dangerous for patients with kidney disease, hypertension, and heart disease such as congestive heart failure.

Finally, the introduction of medications using IV fluids is not reversible. Once the medication or fluids have been injected into the veins, the medication will travel immediately throughout the body. Blood needs only 1 minute to circulate through the body. An IV administration of fluids or medication is systemically distributed in the same amount of time. Even the immediate discontinuation of an injected fluid does *not* prevent body absorption.

The medical assistant must use strict aseptic technique, meet all infection-control standards, continually observe the injection site, and follow the physician's orders exactly. Only with a competent level of education and technical knowledge should any health care professional begin IV therapy or monitor an infusion. The danger to the patient is great, and the ability to evaluate a situation for possible adverse reactions is a necessity before the responsibility of administering IV therapy is accepted.

As with all parenteral administration practices, the health care professional is exposed to needle sticks that may result in the transmission of hepatitis B and HIV viruses and other blood-borne pathogens. Adherence to OSHA guidelines, strict aseptic technique, and the use of personal protective equipment must be followed.

TYPES OF AND REASONS FOR IV THERAPY

In ambulatory care, IV fluids are administered as intermittent infusions to care for an acute condition that does not require hospitalization. IV fluids also are given to maintain fluid intake during illness, reestablish plasma volume, replace electrolyte losses resulting from gastrointestinal diseases, and provide nutrition in patients who cannot consume enough calories daily. Vitamins, minerals, and other nutritional supplements may be added when IV fluids are used to maintain homeostasis. The types of parenteral fluids can contain dextrose, sodium chloride, and other electrolytes.

One simple IV solution is 0.9% sodium chloride, or normal saline. This isotonic solution maintains body fluid levels and does not result in a shift in the fluid in the intracellular, intravascular, and extracellular spaces. IV fluids usually are combined with glucose (for example, dextrose 5% in water [D-5-W] or saline [D-5-NS]) to supply nutritional needs and provide part of the daily caloric requirement. The higher the concentration of dextrose, the more likely the solution will cause a shift in body fluids. Higher concentrations of dextrose (5% or greater) tend to be more characteristic of hypotonic solutions that decrease intravascular fluid loss and increase cellular edema. A third common type of IV fluid is a multiple electrolyte solution such as Ringer's or lactated Ringer's, which contains sodium, potassium, calcium, and chloride ions. Unless dextrose is added to Ringer's solutions, no calories are supplied. Because of the increase in electrolytes, Ringer's solutions are contraindicated in patients with congestive heart failure, renal impairment, and liver disease.

Hypotonic fluids hydrate cells and deplete the amount of fluid in the circulatory system. Fluid moves from the vascular system into the intracellular spaces. The person administering these fluids must remember that a fall in circulating plasma results in lowered blood pressure. For the person who is hypotensive, the use of hypotonic fluids may further lower blood pressure to a dangerous level.

Hypertonic fluids are used to replace electrolytes. Administration causes a shift of extracellular fluids from the interstitial spaces into the plasma for increased blood volumes. These fluids can be used when the extracellular fluids need to be shifted into the plasma, such as with severe edema. These fluids must be given slowly, and the patient must be monitored closely for circulatory overload with symptoms such as shortness of breath, cough, and pitting edema in dependent areas. All IV fluids should be administered with care, but the health care professional should be especially observant with hypertonic solutions because they may result in increased fluids in the blood vessels and circulatory system with resultant complications for the patient.

Isotonic solutions are similar to body fluids and are used to expand the extracellular fluid space. These fluids do not cause the shift of body fluids into other compartments, but circulatory overload is a danger. Isotonic fluids may also dilute the concentration of hemoglobin and lower hematocrit levels when given in large amounts.

Before use, fluids for IV infusion therapy are carefully inspected. The containers are held up to a light to check for clarity and floating precipitates. Any discoloration or precipitate indicates contamination. Only fluids that have not passed the expiration date are used. The date and time of administration are noted and placed on the bag, but not written directly on the bag to prevent puncturing it.

Tables 1 and 2 contain only the infusion fluids most commonly seen in ambulatory care facilities. The figures include parenteral fluid containers in 500 and 1000 mL. Infusion fluids also are available in 50-, 100-, and 250-mL containers. Many different types of parenteral solutions are available. Most physicians in the ambulatory setting use the fluids that have the least chance of causing adverse reactions. For a more acutely, chronically, or critically ill person, the physician may order that drugs, supplements, or fluids be added to the parenteral fluids in specific acute situations. Fat emulsions may also be given intravenously for the patient who needs parenteral nutrition.

EQUIPMENT FOR INFUSION THERAPY

Equipment for administering infusion therapy usually is found in kits that contain the necessary supplies for safe IV access. Each packaged set contains the cannula and needle needed for the injection and IV tubing with the associated attachments to the container of fluids. Each set is individually labeled with the name, description of the equipment, lot number, drops-per-milliliter rate for the chamber and drip orifice, usage description, and manufacturer's name. Each administration set should be carefully chosen by the person starting the infusion to ensure that the kit provides the ordered IV infusion rate and is inspected for maintenance of sterility.

Fluid administration sets come in several types, such as primary administration sets used to provide medications directly into the bloodstream, secondary infusion sets used to add intermittent medications through secondary tubing, and blood administration sets. In most ambulatory care settings, primary administration sets are used for infusion. The patient's condition and physician's order for flow time also are considered in the selection of the desired infusion set. Gravity tubing or infusion pump tubing is used. Primary (standard) sets are available in macrodrip form administering 8 to 20 drops/mL and microdrip form administering 50 to 60 drops/mL (Figure 1). (The microdrip administration set has a smaller drop orifice diameter, so it supplies more drops per milliliter and a slower rate of infusion.) The drip size, or calibration, is clearly marked on the box of the administration set and also in the literature accompanying the set. The macrodrip set, with its large drip size, is more commonly used in adults, and the microdrip or minidrip set is more frequently used when small amounts of fluids are required such as in pediatric patients or with medications that require slow administration.

Tubing varies in length from 60 to 110 inches. The amount of tubing needed for the patient to have some mobility and the placement of the fluids in relation to the patient's position are the determining factors for the length of the tubing used. A sharp spike or piercing tip at the top of the tubing allows the insertion of the tubing into the fluids. When the tubing is inserted into the bag, this spike can perforate the side of the bag, so care must be taken to prevent fluid contamination and to prevent damage to the fluids container. Directly under the spike is a vent, which permits the movement of air to displace the infusing fluids, and the drip chamber, which is a pliable enlarged plastic tube that holds the fluids before infusion. The opening of the drip chamber from the spike contains the drop orifice, which determines the size and shape of the drop of fluids (Figure 2). A flow control clamp compresses the tubing to regulate the rate of infusion and is located on the tubing that descends from the drip chamber (Figure 3). Most clamps are either roller or screw clamps, although the less reliable sliding clamp may also be found, depending on the administration set used in the medical setting. Most tubing has a Luer-Lok connector at the

Text continued on p. 11

Table 1	Fluids for maintaining homeostasis	
Common IV fluid	**Use**	**Contraindications**
Isotonic saline (0.9%)	Replaces sodium losses in conditions such as gastrointestinal fluid loss and burns	Congestive heart failure, pulmonary edema, renal impairment
Isotonic 5% dextrose in water (D-5-W) Hypotonic 10% dextrose in water (D-10-W)	Maintain fluid intake and provide daily caloric needs, acts as peripheral nutrition, does not replace electrolyte deficiencies	Head injuries, added insulin for persons with diabetes mellitus
Isotonic 5% dextrose in 0.3% NaCl	Supplies calories for nutritional needs	No typical contraindications, added insulin for persons with diabetes mellitus
Hypotonic 5% dextrose in 0.9% NaCl	Maintains fluid intake, is maintenance fluid of choice if no electrolytes are needed	No typical contraindications, added insulin for persons with diabetes mellitus
Isotonic Ringer's solution	Replaces electrolytes in concentrations similar to normal plasma levels, contains no calories	Electrolyte replacement unneeded
Isotonic lactated Ringer's solution	Has similar electrolytes as in plasma, is lactated to correct metabolic acidosis, replaces fluid losses from conditions such as diarrhea and burns	Congestive heart failure, renal impairment, liver disease, respiratory alkalosis

Table 2	Advantages and disadvantages of common fluids	
Common solution	**Advantages**	**Disadvantages**
Dextrose in water	Provides carbohydrates, provides nutrition, can be used to treat dehydration	Must be used with care in patients with diabetes
Saline solutions	Provides replacement of extracellular fluids, is used to treat patients with sodium depletion	May provide more sodium and potassium than needed, can lead to circulatory overload
Dextrose in normal saline	Can be used to treat circulatory insufficiency, replaces nutrients and electrolytes, is a hydrating solution	May provide more sodium and potassium than needed, can lead to circulatory overload
Ringer's solution	Acts as a fluid and an electrolyte replacement, is a replenisher after dehydration, is similar to normal saline	Can be incompatible with medications, has no calories, causes sodium retention with subsequent congestive heart failure and renal insufficiency
Lactated Ringer's solution	Acts much like extracellular electrolytes	Has no calories, can be incompatible with medications, can increase sodium levels in person with normal sodium levels

EXAMPLES OF INTRAVENOUS FLUID BAGS AND LABELS

5% dextrose.

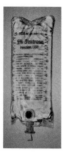

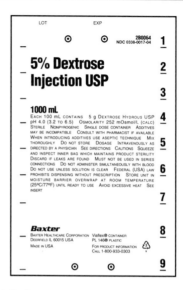

LOT	EXP
⊙	⊙ NDC 0338-0017-04 2B0064 **1**
	2
5% Dextrose	
Injection USP	
	3
1000 mL	
Each 100 mL contains 5 g Dextrose Hydrous USP	**4**
pH 4.0 (3.2 to 6.5) Osmolarity 252 mOsmol/L (calc)	
Sterile Nonpyrogenic Single dose container Additives	
may be incompatible Consult with pharmacist if available	
When introducing additives use aseptic technique Mix	
thoroughly Do not store Dosage Intravenously as	**5**
directed by a physician See directions Cautions Squeeze	
and inspect inner bag which maintains product sterility	
Discard if leaks are found Must not be used in series	
connections Do not administer simultaneously with blood	**6**
Do not use unless solution is clear Federal (USA) law	
prohibits dispensing without prescription Store unit in	
moisture barrier overwrap at room temperature	
(25ºC/77ºF) until ready to use Avoid excessive heat See	
insert	**7**
Baxter	**8**
Baxter Healthcare Corporation Viaflex® container	
Deerfield IL 60015 USA PL 146® plastic	
Made in USA For product information Call 1-800-933-0303	
⊙ ⊙	**9**

From Brown M, Mulholland JM: *Drug calculations: process and problems for clinical practice,* ed 7, St Louis, 2004, Mosby.

Normal saline 0.9%.

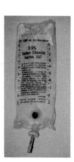

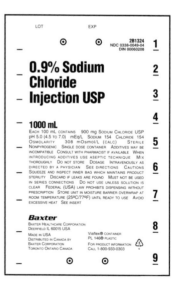

LOT	EXP
⊙	⊙ NDC 0338-0049-04 2B1324 DIN 00060208 **1**
	2
0.9% Sodium	
Chloride	
Injection USP	**3**
	4
1000 mL	
Each 100 mL contains 900 mg Sodium Chloride USP	
pH 5.0 (4.5 to 7.0) mEq/L Sodium 154 Chloride 154	**5**
Osmolarity 308 mOsmol/L (calc) Sterile	
Nonpyrogenic Single dose container Additives may be	
incompatible Consult with pharmacist if available When	
introducing additives use aseptic technique Mix	
thoroughly Do not store Dosage Intravenously as	**6**
directed by a physician See directions Cautions	
Squeeze and inspect inner bag which maintains product	
sterility Discard if leaks are found Must not be used	
in series connections Do not use unless solution is	
clear Federal (USA) law prohibits dispensing without	**7**
prescription Store unit in moisture barrier overwrap at	
room temperature (25ºC/77ºF) until ready to use Avoid	
excessive heat See insert	
Baxter	**8**
Baxter Healthcare Corporation	
Deerfield IL 60015 USA	
Made in USA Viaflex® container	
Distributed in Canada by PL 146® plastic	
Baxter Corporation For product information	
Toronto Ontario Canada Call 1-800-933-0303	
⊙ ⊙	**9**

From Brown M, Mulholland JM: *Drug calculations: process and problems for clinical practice,* ed 7, St Louis, 2004, Mosby.

Continued.

EXAMPLES OF INTRAVENOUS FLUID BAGS AND LABELS—cont'd

Normal saline 0.45%.

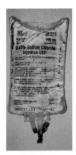

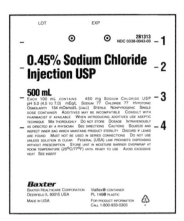

From Brown M, Mulholland JM: *Drug calculations: process and problems for clinical practice,* ed 7, St Louis, 2004, Mosby.

5% dextrose in normal saline.

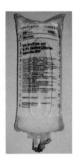

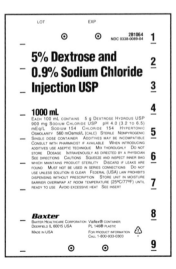

From Brown M, Mulholland JM: *Drug calculations: process and problems for clinical practice,* ed 7, St Louis, 2004, Mosby.

EXAMPLES OF INTRAVENOUS FLUID BAGS AND LABELS—cont'd

5% dextrose in ½ normal saline.

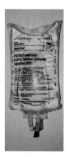

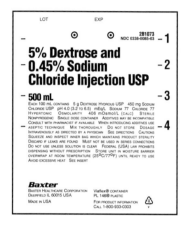

From Brown M, Mulholland JM: *Drug calculations: process and problems for clinical practice,* ed 7, St Louis, 2004, Mosby.

Lactated Ringer's solution.

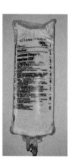

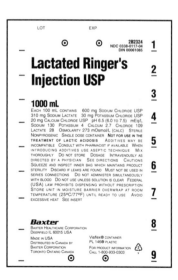

From Brown M, Mulholland JM: *Drug calculations: process and problems for clinical practice,* ed 7, St Louis, 2004, Mosby.

Continued.

EXAMPLES OF INTRAVENOUS FLUID BAGS AND LABELS—cont'd

Lactated Ringer's and 5% dextrose.

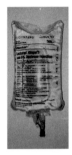

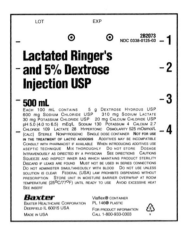

From Brown M, Mulholland JM: *Drug calculations: process and problems for clinical practice,* ed 7, St Louis, 2004, Mosby.

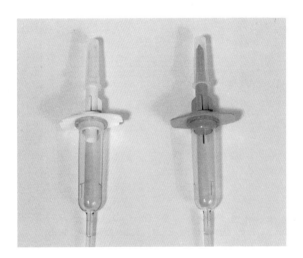

Figure 1 *Left,* IV macrodrip set. *Right,* Microdrip set. (From Leahy JM, Kizilay PE: *Foundations of nursing practice: a nursing process approach,* Philadelphia, 1998, Saunders.)

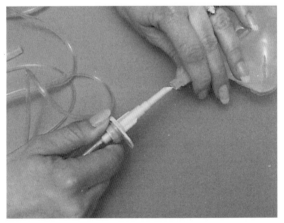

Figure 2 Inserting the spike into the IV fluid bag. (From Perry AG, Potter PA: *Clinical nursing skills and techniques,* ed 6, St Louis, 2006, Mosby.)

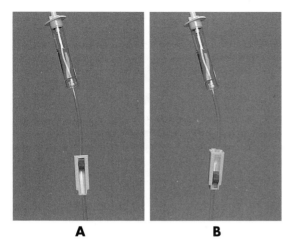

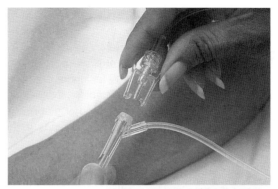

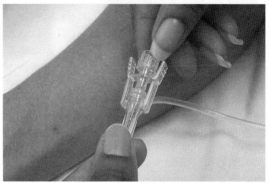

A   **B**

Figure 3 Roller clamp for the regulation of the infusion rate. **A,** Open position, **B,** Closed position. (From Perry AG, Potter PA: *Clinical nursing skills and techniques,* ed 6, St Louis, 2006, Mosby.)

needle to prevent the accidental disconnection of the needle from the tubing and to serve as the attachment of the needle to the tubing. Some tubing has injection ports that act as access points for the addition of other fluids using secondary infusion sets if needed. These ports should ideally be punctured with needleless or needle-protective devices to prevent needle stick injuries and ensure resealing of the ports after use. Needleless systems consist of a blunt-tipped plastic insertion tool and a port for injection that opens on activation and immediately reseals (Figure 4). As with other injectable devices, the shielded needle prevents accidental needle stick injuries by the health care worker by covering the needle after use (Figure 5).

Fluids are most often provided in plastic containers, although glass containers are available. The use of plastic containers prevents breakage and allows stable transport. The containers are relatively light and can be stored in small areas. As fluids are infused, the bag collapses, preventing the need for venting the container. The tubing used for plastic containers does not contain the vent that is necessary with glass containers. Although the safety of these containers usually is easily maintained, each bag should be examined for tears, perforations, and any signs of being unsealed before use.

Figure 4 Example of a needleless protective system. (From Perry AG, Potter PA: *Clinical nursing skills and techniques,* ed 6, St Louis, 2006, Mosby.)

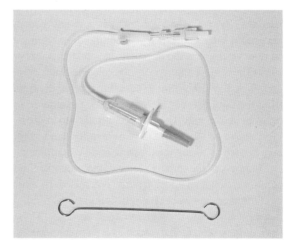

Figure 5 Intravenous equipment, including tubing, drip chamber, spike, tubing, flow-control clamp, and Luer-Lok connector. (From Leahy JM, Kizilay PE: *Foundations of nursing practice: a nursing process approach,* Philadelphia, 1998, Saunders.)

In some ambulatory care settings, a winged-tip (butterfly) needle may be used for short-term infusion therapy, especially after phlebotomy for laboratory testing. Winged-infusion needles are available from size 25 to size 17 and in lengths from 0.5 to 1.0 inch. The tip of the stainless steel needle can puncture the blood vessel wall after placement, causing the risk of infiltration of the fluids if the patient does not remain relatively inactive.

Over-the-needle catheters consist of a needle with a plastic or plasticlike sheath covering the distal point of the needle. The needle, or stylet, is used to inject the vein and guide the catheter. When the catheter is in the vein, a flashback of blood occurs into a chamber behind the catheter hub. The catheter is then threaded off the needle, leaving the softer catheter in place. The catheter needle comes in lengths from 0.5 to 2 inches and gauges of even numbers from 24 to 12. The shortest catheter with the smallest appropriate gauge should be used to deliver the ordered fluids; 22 or 24 gauges are used usually in ambulatory care. The vein must be large enough or the catheter small enough to allow sufficient flow of blood past the injection site to decrease the irritation to the vein wall (Figure 6).

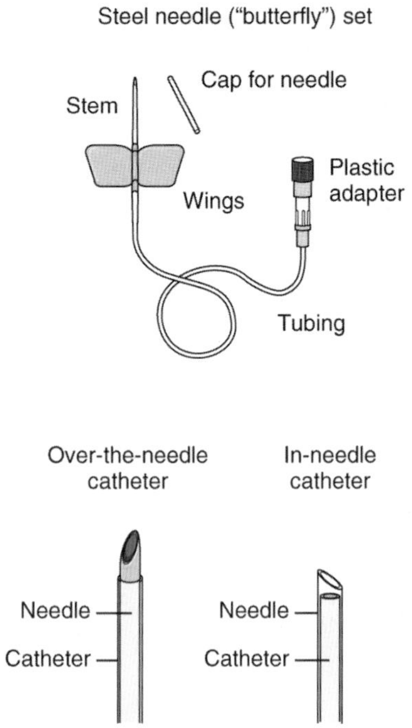

After the venipuncture, the hub of the needle is secured by a dressing to prevent movement in the vein. The choice of the dressing material depends on the needle support for the IV equipment and any patient allergies. Gauze is inexpensive, but the dressing must be removed to view the injection site, and then another sterile dressing is applied. Semipermeable transparent dressings allow moisture to pass through the dressing from the skin, but may be loosened by perspiration or drainage at the site. These especially designed dressings adhere to the skin and minimize the amount of tape needed to secure the dressing and IV equipment.

Clamps on the tubing control the rate of fluid administration if an infusion pump is not used. In some circumstances, an electronic infusion pump is used to deliver the fluids to the highest rate of accuracy. These devices may be stationary, such as a pump attached to an IV pole, or ambulatory, such as a battery-operated pump attached to the patient's clothing. In most cases, controllers on the IV infusion tubing are used as infusion-assist devices that rely on gravity for the

Figure 6 Equipment for starting short-term peripheral IV infusions: winged-infusion needle and over-the-needle catheter. (From Leahy JM, Kizilay PE: *Foundations of nursing practice: a nursing process approach,* Philadelphia, 1998, Saunders.)

proper rate of fluid administration. A drop-sensor placed on the drip chamber also is used with controllers to indicate the flow of fluids. The controller monitors the infusion and beeps to alert the patient and health care professionals when flow is interrupted. Controllers do not push fluids into the patient but rather allow monitoring of fluid infusion. The accuracy of this type of equipment depends on drops being uniform.

The specific equipment needed for infusion therapy varies among offices and patients. The health care professional must know which equipment best suits the patient's condition and must follow the physician's order to provide the ordered fluids with the least discomfort for the patient.

CALCULATION OF IV FLOW RATES

The physician orders the flow rate of fluids. To calculate the rate of infiltration, the medical assistant must know the volume of fluid to be infused, the length of time for the infusion as ordered by the physician, and the manufacturer's drop rate (number of drops per milliliter). The tubing may be microdrip or macrodrip, as previously described, and the manufacturer provides the information in drops per milliliter on the packaging for the drop rate needed in each calculation to meet the physician's order.

The first step in calculating the rate of infiltration requires the calculation of the total volume of fluid to be administered in an hour. The following formula is used:

$$\frac{\text{Total volume to be infused}}{\text{Time in total hours}} = \text{Volume per hour}$$

Then the drop-per-minute (gtt/min) rate is calculated using the following formula:

$$\frac{\text{Volume to infuse per hour} \times \text{drops/mL (on tubing box)}}{60 \text{ min (1 hr)}}$$

$$= \text{gtt/min}$$

EXAMPLE:

The physician orders 1000 mL of D-5-W to be infused over 6 hours. The tubing reads 20 mL/min.

The amount to be infused in an hour is determined as follows:

$$\frac{1000 \text{ mL}}{6 \text{ hr}} = \text{Volume per hour}$$

The volume per hour is 167 gtt/mL.

$$\frac{167 \text{ mL} \times 20 \text{ mL}}{60 \text{ min}} = \text{gtt/min}$$

$$\frac{3340}{60} = \text{gtt/min}$$

The volume to be given is 56 gtt/min.

With this order, the drip rate is set at 56 mL/min. The flow rate should be monitored to ensure that this rate remains correct over the time of the entire infusion.

SCREENING BEFORE IV ADMINISTRATION

Before ordering an IV infusion, the physician performs a baseline screening of the patient. A medical assistant usually assists. An accurate medical history taken before infusion allows health care workers to determine whether changes have occurred in the patient's condition during infusion therapy. The history should include both medical conditions and family history; this information is documented for future reference during the infusion.

A clinical screening is equally important. The patient's body weight during therapy is compared with the baseline weight; rapid changes usually indicate fluid loss or gain. A total of 1 pound of body weight is approximately 500 mL of fluids.

The concentration of urine is determined during the initial screening; a urinalysis allows the medical team to assess the patient's hydration level. In diuresis (the increased formation and excretion of urine), low specific gravity and dilution of urine occur; in dehydration, a higher specific gravity or urine concentration occurs, necessitating hydration therapy. Checking the physical properties, such as color, specific gravity and odor, of the urine provides this information.

Vital signs also are taken and recorded before, during, and after therapy according to the policy of the health care institution. Electrolyte changes and fluid loss may cause hypotension, especially during postural changes, and fluid gain may increase blood pressure and cause breathing difficulties.

Behavioral changes, such as restlessness and apprehension, may indicate fluid deficit. Increased irritability, disorientation, and mental confusion may result from fluid loss or electrolyte imbalance. Although screening for these signs is not legally indicated, such signs should be documented before fluid administration; belligerence, disorientation, and lethargy should also be documented.

SCREENING DURING IV INFUSION

The health care worker should screen frequently for complications so that early interventions can occur. Complications may be either local or systemic and include infiltration, phlebitis, hematoma, circulatory system overload, and local infection. Problems with equipment can also occur.

Infiltration of fluids is a common local complication. The signs of infiltration include a slowing or stopping of fluid infusion, tissue induration, and swelling around the injection site with tissue remaining cool to the touch. (An alarm sounds if infiltration occurs with an infusion device.) If it does occur, the infusion site is changed, and the affected arm is elevated and covered with warm compresses. Infiltration is prevented by observing the IV site at least every hour and anchoring the tubing to prevent movement.

Although not common in ambulatory care, phlebitis, an inflammation of the veins, can occur, especially if fluids are given on successive days. Phlebitis is indicated by at least two of the following: redness, pain, swelling, and warmth at the site. Inflammation may cause the vein to feel like a cord. If phlebitis occurs, the infusion site should be moved, and warm compresses should be applied to the area of induration and redness.

Nicking of the vein during venipuncture, application of a tourniquet above the area of a previously attempted venipuncture site, or a leaky vein from frequent injections may cause a hematoma, especially in those who bruise easily. Discoloration of the skin, swelling, and discomfort are typical signs. Careful venipuncture technique and the correct placement of the tourniquet prevent this complication.

If a local infection occurs at the venipuncture site, the site and the catheter, if present, should be cultured. Redness and a purulent exudate are common signs of infection. The patient may also have a fever and an elevated white blood cell count. The infusion should be stopped and restarted, if appropriate, and the infected site is covered with sterile dressings. The best prevention is good aseptic technique at the time of venipuncture and throughout infusion.

Too-rapid infusion of IV fluids causes circulatory system overload. If overload occurs, the physician is notified immediately, and vital signs are taken. The patient is checked for shortness of breath, pitting edema, a rise in blood pressure, and other signs of cardiac problems. Checking flow rate calculations at least twice before starting the infusion can help prevent this complication. Controllers or infusion devices should be used in patients at greatest risk. Time-tapes applied to the fluid container indicate the amount of fluid that should be administered

each hour. These tapes, which easily indicate whether the fluids are infusing too slowly or rapidly, are attached to the fluid container for quick evaluation and adjustment, as needed, of the infusion rate. It is very important that all infusion rates be calculated twice and then checked by another medical professional if any questions of accuracy are present.

If the infusion becomes sluggish, the tubing should be observed for kinking or another obstruction; the patient also could be lying on the tubing. If correcting these problems does not correct the flow rate, the injection site may need to be repositioned or relocated.

If the tubing is not tightly attached to the needle, leaking may occur at the needle-tubing junction. If the tubing is contaminated because of the leak, it must be changed. The use of Luer-Lok devices and proper connection of the tubing to the needle should prevent this potential problem because the needle is locked into place.

An obstructed IV line may need to be flushed. This should be done *only* by a professional knowledgeable in the technique. The flush should not be forced; the infusion site should be changed if minimal pressure fails to reopen the IV line.

The administration of cold IV fluids causes venous spasm. There is a sharp pain along the length of the vein, and the infusion may slow. Thus fluids should be at room temperature when they are administered.

LEGAL AND ETHICAL ISSUES

The physician is legally responsible for the actions of the unlicensed professional following his or her orders, but the medical assistant does have the legal responsibility for ensuring that no procedure is attempted for which he or she has no educational or technical background. State medical practice acts define which procedures the medical assistant can perform, and the medical assistant must always be aware of the changes legislated in each state and must ensure that his or her actions are in compliance with the laws. Because states continuously change the medical assistant's scope of practice, the person starting IV infusions must keep abreast of the statues of the state of practice. Ignorance of the law is not an acceptable defense when prohibited procedures are performed or when life-threatening critical errors occur.

Because there is an increasing need for medical assistants to perform more advanced procedures in ambulatory care settings, these health care professionals also are being placed in situations that require ethical decision-making. Because ethical decisions are essentially moral decisions, they are individual and can change with each professional situation. The health care worker must decide on the "right" course by relying on his or her own educational and technical background.

IV infusion is a highly technical skill that requires a knowledge base that is also skilled. The exact procedure for performing the initiation of IV fluids is a very similar to that for performing a venipuncture, but the introduction of fluids or medications into the veins has greater potential for harm. The ethical decisions are therefore much harder to make and must be made with patient safety in the forefront.

The fact that a procedure is legally within the scope of practice in a specific geographical area does not necessarily mean that it should be performed by all personnel who can legally perform it. Critical thinking skills, as well as knowledge of technique and screening, are essential for patient safety, and the medical assistant must be proficient and knowledgeable in these areas before performing IV initiation and infusion therapy. The ethical responsibility of acknowledging limitations in technical skills and knowledge belongs solely to the person asked to perform the task; the medical assistant must make the ethical decision about whether the task is within her or his scope of practice.

Because a task is legal does not necessarily mean that it is ethical. The health care professional should always ask, "Is this a task that I would do to myself if I could? Would I feel comfortable if I were the patient during this procedure? Are my knowledge and technical base adequate for patient safety?" The medical assistant should know all aspects of the procedure to be performed. He or she also should know the adverse reactions and the treatment of each.

PREPARING THE SITE FOR INITIATION OF IV THERAPY

Purpose

To prepare for venipuncture using the supplies for the infusion of IV fluids

Conditions

Using the following, prepare the site for and initiate IV therapy: a physician's order for the IV therapy containing the IV fluids to be used and the length of the infusion, proper IV fluids as ordered by the physician, administration kit with the correct drop orifice for the physician's order, an IV pole, a drop-control device as indicated, gloves, cleansing and antiseptic skin preparations, dressings, tape (appropriate for the patient's skin condition and possible allergies), a tourniquet, a rigid biohazard container, a biohazardous waste container, 2 × 2 or 4 × 4 sterile gauze sponges, a transparent dressing for the injection site, and an arm board if indicated.

Standard

Passing this procedure requires that it be completed within ____ minutes at an accuracy rate of ____%.

Step 1

Identify the patient. Explain the procedure and ask the patient whether he or she has questions. Wash the hands and perform baseline patient screening. Take vital signs and document them. Place the patient in a comfortable position.

Rationale: Identification of the patient ensures that the correct patient is receiving the fluids. Explanation of the procedure ensures cooperation of the patient and implies that consent has been obtained. Washing the hands using standards set by the Occupational Safety and Health Administration is necessary for infection control. Screening the patient's condition provides a baseline for determining whether complications or adverse reactions have occurred. Documentation is necessary for registering the care provided.

Step 2

In the preparation area, assemble the needed supplies and check for expiration dates and for any indications of contamination. Always compare the supplies to the physician's order, using the seven rights of medication administration at the three times that medications should be checked. Open the sterile packages using proper aseptic technique. Prepare the fluids for injection by removing the cover of the fluids, the cover of the spike insertion site, and the spike on the tubing. Insert the spike into the fluids container (see Figure 2).

Rationale: Preparations for patient care, especially when giving medications, should be accomplished in a quiet area to prevent errors. The needed supplies and equipment must not be out of date and must match the physician's order to prevent errors. All fluids should be checked for currency of date and for signs of contamination. If the date of use has expired or if contamination is obvious, the fluids should not be used. Proper opening of sterile infusion sets and fluids maintains sterility and prevents potential contamination of the fluids and tubing. The spike must remain sterile and should be placed within the fluid bag to allow for the removal of fluids from the bag for administration to the patient.

Step 3

Adjust the roller clamp on the tubing to about 1 to 2 inches below the drip chamber. Allow fluids to fill the drip chamber until it is approximately half full by gently compressing the chamber with the fingers (Figure 7). With the roller clamp open, remove the cap of the infusion tubing and allow fluids to travel from the drip chamber through the tubing to the needle adapter. Clamp the tubing when the tubing is filled, and replace the protector cap on the end of the tubing with the appropriate needle/catheter, taking care to maintain the sterility of the tip. Flick the tubing to remove air bubbles (Figure 8).

Rationale: The roller clamp should be in a position that allows for a more accurate control of the flow rate and ease of viewing. The drip chamber and

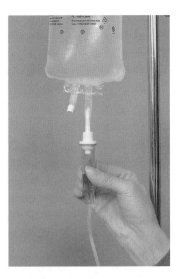

Figure 7 (From Perry AG, Potter PA: *Clinical nursing skills and techniques,* ed 6, St Louis, 2006, Mosby.)

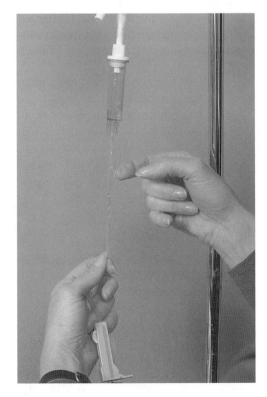

Figure 8 (From Perry AG, Potter PA: *Clinical nursing skills and techniques,* ed 6, St Louis, 2006, Mosby.)

tubing should be filled to prevent the flow of air into the vein, but it is not filled over half full so that the flow of drops into the chamber can be observed and the drip rate can be watched. Filling the tubing ensures that air has been removed from the administration set to prevent air emboli. Replacing the protector cap with the needle maintains solution sterility and prepares the fluids for infusion.

Step 4

Return to the procedure area with the prepared equipment. Apply disposable gloves and other personal protective equipment as appropriate. Inspect the arm for an injection site. Apply a tourniquet approximately 4 inches above the selected site, being careful to apply it with adequate but not tight pressure. Check for a radial pulse to be sure the circulation to the area has not been obstructed. Look for a vein that is sufficiently large for needle or catheter placement, preferably on the nondominant side at a distal site that does not interfere with activities of daily living (Figure 9).

Rationale: Personal protective equipment is necessary for infection control and for the protection of the person performing the task. The patient's arm should be inspected for the best possible site for needle insertion; areas where skin is not intact and areas where the integrity of the arm is at risk are avoided. The tourniquet should not be so tight that it impedes arterial blood flow. The site should be comfortable for the patient and allow some movement for personal care. Placement in more distal areas of the arm allows more proximal areas to be used if additional IV therapy is needed. The vein should be large enough to allow venous flow after venipuncture.

Step 5

Select a well-dilated vein (Figure 10). If the tourniquet has been in place over 2 minutes, release, wait a minute, and reapply.

Rationale: A large visible vein is the best choice for venipuncture. If the tourniquet has been in place for over 2 minutes, blood flow must be restored; then venipuncture process is continued.

Step 6

Position the adapter end on a sterile gauze or towel near the venipuncture site. Reapply the tourniquet and prepare the site according to office policy (Figure 11). If the site needs cleansing, use soap and water followed by either povidone-iodine or 70% alcohol in a circular motion. Allow the site to dry and do not touch it. Prepare two or three strips of tape or a transparent dressing; place the dressing materials near the injection site.

Rationale: The adapter should be in close proximity to the site for performing venipuncture. The site must be cleansed using the preferred agent as stated in office policy to maintain asepsis and infection control. Allowing the area to dry prevents patient discomfort.

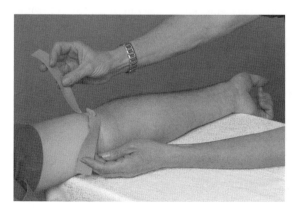

Figure 9 (From Perry AG, Potter PA: *Clinical nursing skills and techniques,* ed 6, St Louis, 2006, Mosby.)

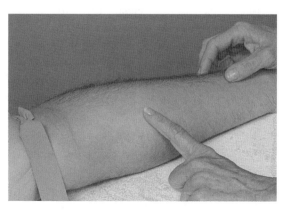

Figure 10 (From Perry AG, Potter PA: *Clinical nursing skills and techniques,* ed 6, St Louis, 2006, Mosby.)

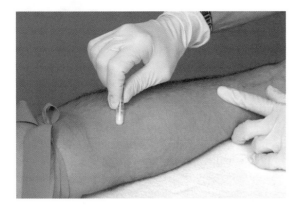

Figure 11 (From Perry AG, Potter PA: *Clinical nursing skills and techniques,* ed 6, St Louis, 2006, Mosby.)

Touching would contaminate the cleansed area. Dressing materials should be readily available.

Step 7

Ask the patient to open and close his or her fist several times to distend the veins. Anchor the vein by placing the thumb over it and applying upward pressure to make the skin taut (Figure 12). Tell the patient that a sharp, quick stick will occur. Insert the needle distal and parallel to the vein at a 20- to 30-degree angle to the skin using either a winged-infusion set, an over-the needle catheter, or other equipment as preferred by the office of employment. Observe for a flashback of blood into either the tubing of the winged-infusion set or into the flashback chamber of the over-the-needle catheter (Figure 13). Advance the catheter or needle approximately 1/4 to 1/2 inch into the vein, using the dominant hand to push the catheter off the needle and the nondominant hand to hold the flashback chamber (Figure 14). The catheter should be advanced to the hub. Do not reinsert the stylet once it is loosened.

Rationale: Opening and closing the fist distends the vein for easier insertion. Anchoring prevents movement of the vein during injection. The needle must be inserted distal to the vein at an angle of 20 to 30 degrees to prevent puncturing the posterior wall of the vein. If the vein is punctured, a flashback of blood occurs, and the needle or catheter should be advanced into the vein for stabilization. Reinsertion of the stylet could cause breakage of the catheter in the vein.

Step 8

Stabilize the catheter and needle with one hand and loosen the tourniquet with the other. If the catheter is used, cover the stylet with the safety cap as it is removed. Keep the needle stable and dispose of the stylet in a rigid biohazard container. Connect the IV tubing to the hub of the needle or the catheter (Figure 15). Secure the hub with either tape or a transparent dressing as per office policy. If tape is used, place one small strip with the sticky side toward the hub and adhere it to the opposite side of the hub. Repeat with the other end of the tape in a cross-over fashion (Figure 16). If nontransparent tape is used, avoid placing it directly over the insertion site. If a transparent dressing is used, remove the backing and apply one edge; smooth the dressing while

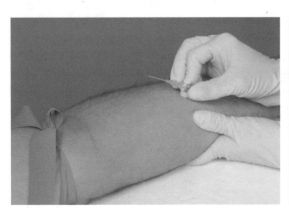

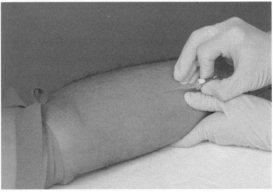

Figure 12 (From Perry AG, Potter PA: *Clinical nursing skills and techniques,* ed 6, St Louis, 2006, Mosby.)

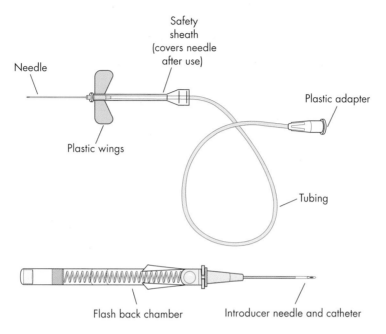

Figure 13 (From Perry AG, Potter PA: *Clinical nursing skills and techniques,* ed 6, St Louis, 2006, Mosby.)

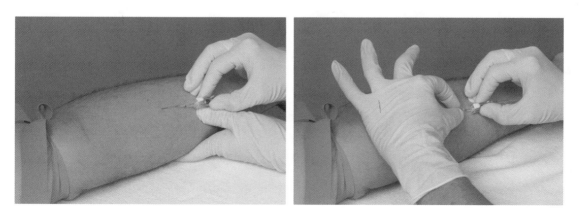

Figure 14 (From Perry AG, Potter PA: *Clinical nursing skills and techniques,* ed 6, St Louis, 2006, Mosby.)

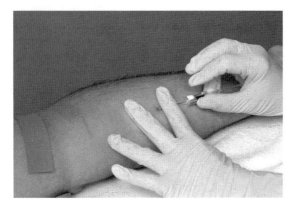

Figure 15 (From Perry AG, Potter PA: *Clinical nursing skills and techniques,* ed 6, St Louis, 2006, Mosby.)

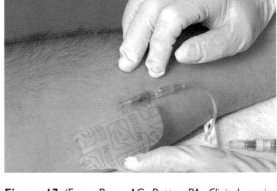

Figure 17 (From Perry AG, Potter PA: *Clinical nursing skills and techniques,* ed 6, St Louis, 2006, Mosby.)

applying it over the site (Figure 17). Open the roller clamp and adjust it to the flow rate ordered by the physician and properly calculated. Make a small loop in the tubing near the insertion site and secure it over the dressing with tape.

Rationale: Stabilization of the needle is essential for preventing accidental dislodgment of the catheter or needle. Covering the stylet on removal prevents personnel injury. Any materials that have come in contact with blood must be disposed of in a rigid biohazard container. The hub must be secured and the tubing looped to prevent dislodgment or damage to the vein. Placing the tape over the dressing prevents further skin irritation.

Step 9

Remove the gloves, sanitize the hands as appropriate, and document the procedure, recording the size of the catheter or winged-infusion set used and the location of the injection site. Document the type of fluids administered, the flow rate, and the patient's reaction to the procedure. Also document any adverse reactions or other information, such as vital signs. Inform the physician of any changes in the patient's condition.

Rationale: Removing the gloves and sanitizing the hands is essential for infection control. No procedure is complete until it is documented.

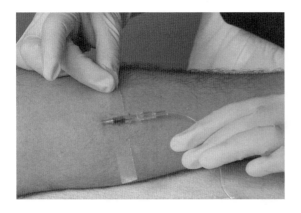

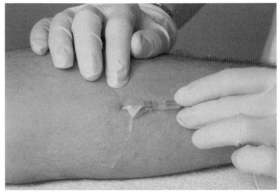

Figure 16 (From Perry AG, Potter PA: *Clinical nursing skills and techniques,* ed 6, St Louis, 2006, Mosby.)

QUESTIONS

1. Why is it important for the medical assistant to use the fluids as ordered by the physician?
2. What is the difference among hypotonic, isotonic, and hypertonic solutions? How do these affect the movement of fluids in the body?
3. What are the three basic types of IV therapy?
4. What are the two types of drip chambers found on IV tubing? Why are they important?
5. Why is urinalysis indicated before IV therapy?
6. Why is it important to carefully calculate the infusion rate for IV therapy?
7. Why is it important to take baseline vital signs when preparing a patient for IV therapy?
8. What are some of the reasons for IV infusion therapy in ambulatory care facilities?
9. Why are both medical and surgical asepsis necessary for IV therapy?
10. What are the legal and ethical implications for the medical assistant who initiates IV therapy?

ANSWERS

1. *Why is it important for the medical assistant to use the fluids as ordered by the physician?* Because the body responds differently to various types of IV fluids, the physician carefully chooses the fluids to be administered. Therefore the medical assistant must be careful that the fluids used are the fluids ordered. Just as with any other physician's order, the order for IV therapy must be followed exactly.
2. *What is the difference among hypotonic, isotonic, and hypertonic solutions? How do these affect the movement of fluids in the body?* Isotonic solutions bathe the body tissues without causing a change of fluids in the cells. Hypertonic solutions move fluids across a semipermeable membrane out of cells, and hypotonic solutions cause the flow of fluids across the membrane into cells.
3. *What are the three basic types of IV therapy?* IV therapy is used for the maintenance, replacement, and restoration of fluids.
4. *What are the two types of drip chambers found on IV tubing? Why are they important?* Drip chambers are available as macrodrip sets that administer 8 to 20 drops/mL and microdrip sets that administer 50 to 60 drops/mL. The medical assistant must choose the correct infusion set with the correct drop size for correct calibration for administration of the fluids.
5. *Why is urinalysis indicated before IV therapy?* Urinalysis allows the hydration level of the patient to be evaluated.
6. *Why is it important to carefully calculate the infusion rate for IV therapy?* Cardiac overload is an increase in the fluid levels of the blood caused by the shift of fluids from the extracellular tissues into the circulating plasma. Because the fluid levels are increased during overload, the heart must work harder to pump blood. A high rate of infusion increases body fluid levels and has a direct effect on the body's ability to circulate the fluids. Physiologically, the body responds to the rate of infusion.
7. *Why is it important to take baseline vital signs when preparing a patient for IV therapy?* Baseline vital signs provide clues about the patient's condition at the start of IV therapy. Vital signs taken during the infusion indicate changes in the patient's vascular condition.
8. *What are some of the reasons for IV infusion therapy in ambulatory care facilities?* IV therapy may be given for any of the three reasons for IV therapy. In most cases, short-term IV therapy is used to rehydrate the patient after severe nausea, vomiting, dehydration, and diarrhea.

9. *Why are both medical and surgical asepsis necessary for IV therapy?* One of the dangers of IV infusion is infection caused by poor aseptic technique. Using medical asepsis for personal cleansing and for care of the patient's skin during venipuncture, as well as maintaining sterile technique during the infusion, is necessary for preventing infection.

10. *What are the legal and ethical implications for the medical assistant who initiates IV therapy?* Legally the medical assistant must perform any procedure following the medical practice act of the state of practice. Ethically, the medical assistant should know all aspects of the procedure that is to be performed. He or she should also know adverse reactions and their treatment. The medical assistant should never participate in any procedure that he or she is not technically prepared to perform and has the knowledge base required for patient safety.

BIBLIOGRAPHY

Brown M, Mulholland JM: *Drug calculations: process and problems for clinical practice,* ed 7, St Louis, 2004, Mosby.

Elkin MK, Perry AG, Potter PA: *Nursing interventions and clinical skills,* ed 3, St Louis, 2004, Mosby.

Fulcher EM, Soto CD, Fulcher RM: *Pharmacology: principles and applications,* Philadelphia, 2003, Saunders.

Leahy JM, Kizilay PE: *Foundations of nursing practice: a nursing process approach,* Philadelphia, 1998, Saunders.

Macklin D, Chernecky C: *Real world nursing survival guide: IV therapy,* Philadelphia, 2004, Saunders.

Otto S: *Intravenous therapy,* ed 4, St. Louis, 2001, Mosby.

Perry AG, Potter PA: *Clinical nursing skills and techniques,* ed 6, St Louis, 2006, Mosby.